T0837614

INTRODUCTION

As Muslims, we are encouraged to take care of our bodies and maintain good health. However, finding reliable information on fitness and nutrition within an Islamic context can be challenging. That's why I, Musa Murad, have written this book.

I am not a certified fitness expert, nutritionist, or Islamic scholar. But I am a practicing Muslim who believes in the importance of incorporating Islamic values and principles into all aspects of my life, including my health and fitness routine. Through extensive research of Islamic sources such as the Quran, Hadith, and Sunnah, I have gained a wealth of knowledge on how to live a healthy lifestyle while adhering to Islamic teachings.

In this book, I will share with you the wisdom and guidance of the Islamic faith as it relates to fitness and nutrition. I have personally applied the Sunnah ways of fitness in my own life and have seen significant positive effects on my health. It is my hope that by sharing my experiences and knowledge, I can help my fellow Muslims lead healthier, more fulfilling lives, in accordance with the teachings of Islam.

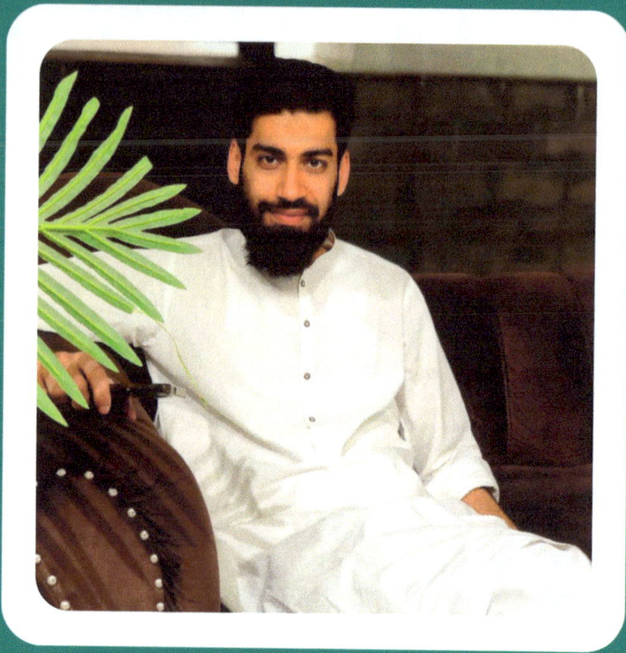

MUSA MURAD

ABOUT THE AUTHOR

Musa Murad is a Muslim who has gained knowledge and experience in physical fitness and nutrition through his personal life and learning from Quran, Hadith, and the Sunnah of Prophet Muhammad (PBUH). He is not a certified Islamic scholar or professional fitness trainer or nutritionist, but his passion lies in guiding fellow Muslims to achieve a healthier lifestyle and a stronger connection with Allah through his e-book. The book serves as a valuable resource for anyone seeking guidance on physical fitness and nutrition in the context of Islam, accessible on any digital device for easy reading.

WHY I WROTE THIS BOOK

As a believer who testifies that there is no deity but Allah and that Muhammad is His messenger, I felt compelled to share my experiences and knowledge on the significance of physical fitness and proper nutrition in Islam. While I am not a certified Islamic scholar, physical fitness expert, or nutritionist, I have gained insight and understanding from the Quran, Hadith, and Sunnah of Prophet Muhammad (PBUH) to lead a healthier lifestyle and strengthen my relationship with Allah. By applying the Sunnah ways of fitness and nutrition in my daily life, I have witnessed the positive effects on my health and well-being. Through this book, I hope to inspire and guide fellow Muslims on their journey towards a healthier lifestyle, while staying true to their faith.

OVERVIEW OF THE BOOK'S CONTENT

The book is structured into nine chapters, each of which explores a different aspect of physical fitness in the context of Islam. Here's a breakdown of the chapters:

Chapter 1: Introduction:
This chapter provides an overview of the importance of physical fitness in Islam, and the book's content and structure.

Chapter 2: Quranic and Hadith-based Principles for Physical Fitness:
This chapter explores the Quranic and Hadith-based principles for physical fitness, highlighting the importance of maintaining good health and taking care of our bodies.

Chapter 3: Diet and Nutrition in Islam:
This chapter discusses the Islamic principles of healthy eating and moderation, as well as the benefits of a balanced diet for physical fitness.

Chapter 4: Exercise and Fitness in Islam:
This chapter delves into the different types of exercises that are permissible in Islam, and the benefits of regular exercise for physical fitness and overall health.

Chapter 5: Fitness of Kids in Islam:
This chapter explores the importance of physical fitness for kids in Islam, and provides guidance on physical activities and exercises that are appropriate and beneficial for children.

Chapter 6: Mental Health and Well-being in Islam:
This chapter discusses the importance of mental health in Islam, and the ways in which we can promote relaxation and stress management through Islamic principles.

Chapter 7: Islam and Sports:
This chapter looks at the history of sports in Islam, and how Islam encourages physical activity and sports.

Chapter 8: Physical Fitness for Women in Islam:
This chapter explores physical fitness for Muslim women, discussing the Islamic principles of modesty and appropriate physical activities for women.

Chapter 9: Conclusion
This chapter summarizes the key principles and takeaways from the book, and emphasizes the importance of physical fitness in the context of Islam.

Overall, "Physical Fitness with Islam" offers a comprehensive guide to physical fitness that is grounded in Islamic principles, and provides practical tips and guidance for readers looking to improve their physical fitness and well-being.

CONTENTS

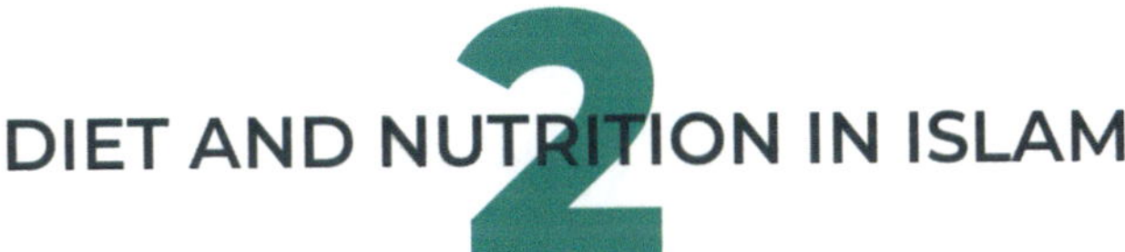

QURANIC AND HADITH-BASED PRINCIPLES
FOR PHYSICAL FITNESS

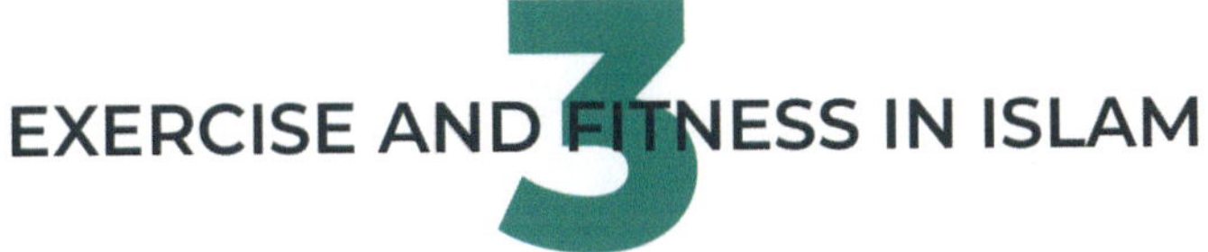

DIET AND NUTRITION IN ISLAM

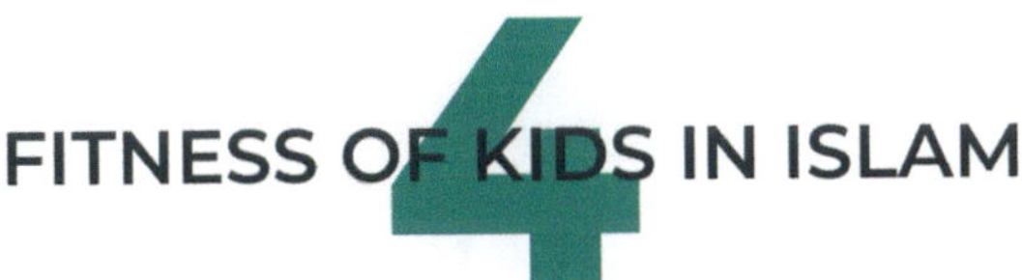

EXERCISE AND FITNESS IN ISLAM

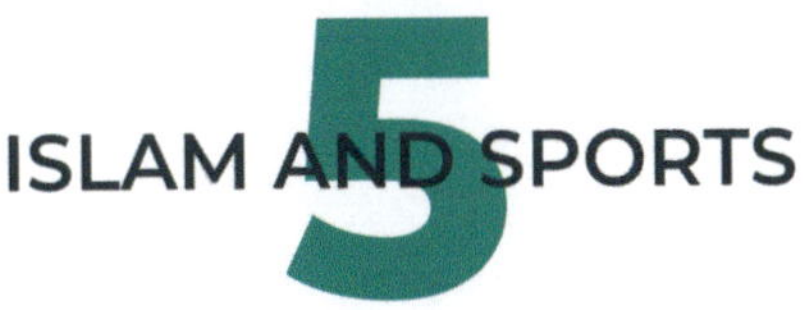

FITNESS OF KIDS IN ISLAM

ISLAM AND SPORTS

QURANIC AND HADITH-BASED PRINCIPLES FOR PHYSICAL FITNESS

Physical fitness and good health are important aspects of our lives as Muslims. In Islam, maintaining good health is considered to be a religious obligation, and taking care of our bodies is seen as a means of showing gratitude to Allah (SWT) for the blessings He has bestowed upon us.

The Quran and Hadith provide us with valuable guidance on the principles of physical fitness. For instance, the Quran says: "And eat and drink but waste not in extravagance, certainly He (Allah) likes not those who waste in extravagance" (Quran 7:31). This verse emphasizes the importance of moderation in our eating and drinking habits, and encourages us to avoid overindulgence.

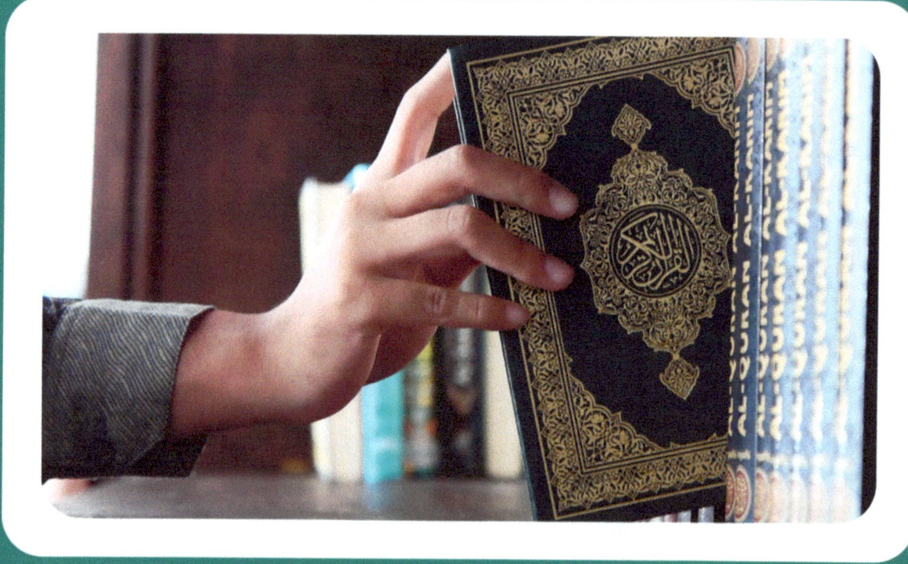

Similarly, the Prophet Muhammad (PBUH) emphasized the importance of physical fitness and encouraged Muslims to engage in physical activities. He said: "A strong believer is better and more beloved to Allah than a weak one" (Sahih Muslim). This Hadith highlights the importance of physical strength and fitness, and encourages Muslims to work towards improving their physical health.

In addition, the Quran emphasizes the importance of taking care of our bodies, which are considered to be a trust from Allah (SWT). The Prophet Muhammad (PBUH) also taught us to treat our bodies with respect and care, saying: "Your body has a right over you" (Sahih Bukhari).

Moreover, Islam encourages us to lead a balanced and healthy lifestyle. This includes not only taking care of our physical health, but also our mental and spiritual well-being. The Quran says: "O ye who believe! Eat of the good things that We have provided for you, and be grateful to Allah, if it is Him ye worship" (Quran 2:172). This verse highlights the importance of eating healthy and nutritious food, and being grateful to Allah (SWT) for the blessings of food and health.

In conclusion, this chapter emphasizes the importance of physical fitness in Islam, and highlights the Quranic and Hadith-based principles that guide us towards maintaining good health and taking care of our bodies. By following these principles, we can improve our physical health, mental well-being, and spiritual connection with Allah (SWT).

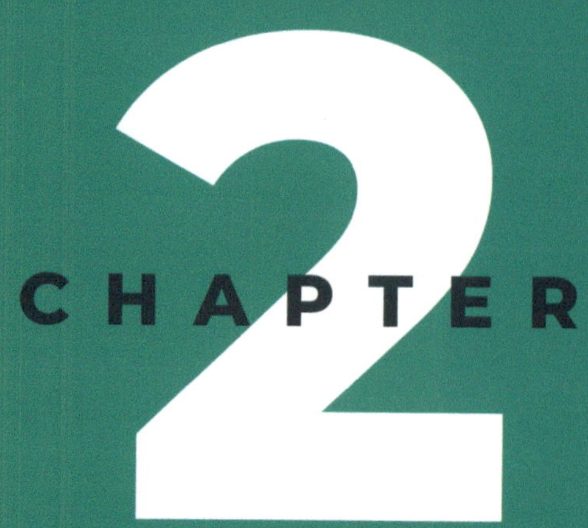

DIET AND NUTRITION IN ISLAM

Diet and nutrition are important components of a healthy lifestyle, and Islam places great emphasis on the importance of a balanced and healthy diet for physical and spiritual well-being. The Quran and Hadith provide guidance on healthy eating habits, highlighting the importance of moderation, consuming nutritious foods, and avoiding excess.

The Islamic principle of moderation is reflected in the Quranic verse that states, "Eat of the good things We have provided for your sustenance, but commit no excess therein, lest My wrath should justly descend on you" (Quran 20:81). This verse emphasizes the importance of consuming food in moderation and avoiding overeating or indulging in unhealthy foods.

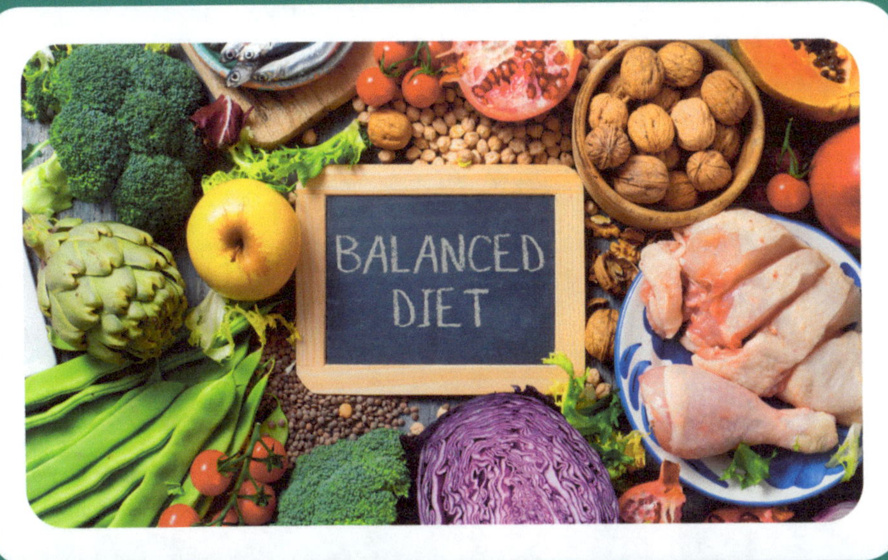

Islam also emphasizes the importance of consuming healthy and nutritious food. The Prophet Muhammad (PBUH) said, "A strong believer is better and more beloved to Allah than a weak one, though both are good. Strive for that which will benefit you, seek the help of Allah, and do not feel helpless. If anything befalls you, do not say, 'If only I had done such and such,' but rather say, 'Allah decrees and what He wills, He does'" (Sahih Muslim). This Hadith highlights the importance of consuming a balanced diet that includes a variety of healthy foods to maintain good physical health and strength.

Islamic principles also encourage the consumption of certain foods and discourage the consumption of others. For example, the Quran promotes the consumption of fruits and vegetables, as well as grains and lean meats. The Prophet Muhammad (PBUH) encouraged the consumption of dates and honey, which are known to have numerous health benefits.

The concept of halal and haram foods also plays a role in healthy eating habits. Halal foods are those that are permissible according to Islamic dietary laws, while haram foods are those that are prohibited. By consuming only halal foods, Muslims can ensure that they are consuming healthy and clean foods.

Prophet Muhammad (PBUH) was a model of healthy eating habits. He ate in moderation, consumed a variety of healthy foods, and avoided overeating or indulging in unhealthy foods. In times of scarcity, he would often survive on dates and water, and in times of abundance, he would share his food with others and give to those in need. His diet consisted of simple, wholesome foods that provided him with the necessary nutrients to maintain his physical health and well-being.

Prophet Muhammad (PBUH) remained humble and thankful to Allah, even in times of hardship or scarcity. He trusted in Allah's provisions and was content with whatever Allah provided him. Allah nourished him with less food, and he remained healthy and in good physical shape. His perfect body shape and health are a testament to his healthy eating habits and his trust in Allah.

In conclusion, a balanced and healthy diet is an essential component of physical and spiritual well-being in Islam. By following Islamic principles of moderation, consuming a variety of healthy foods, and avoiding haram foods, Muslims can maintain physical fitness, improve their health, and fulfill their religious obligations. Prophet Muhammad (PBUH) is a model for healthy eating habits, and his diet consisted of simple, wholesome foods that provided him with the necessary nutrients to maintain his physical health and well-being, even in times of scarcity. His humility and trust in Allah are an example for all Muslims to follow.

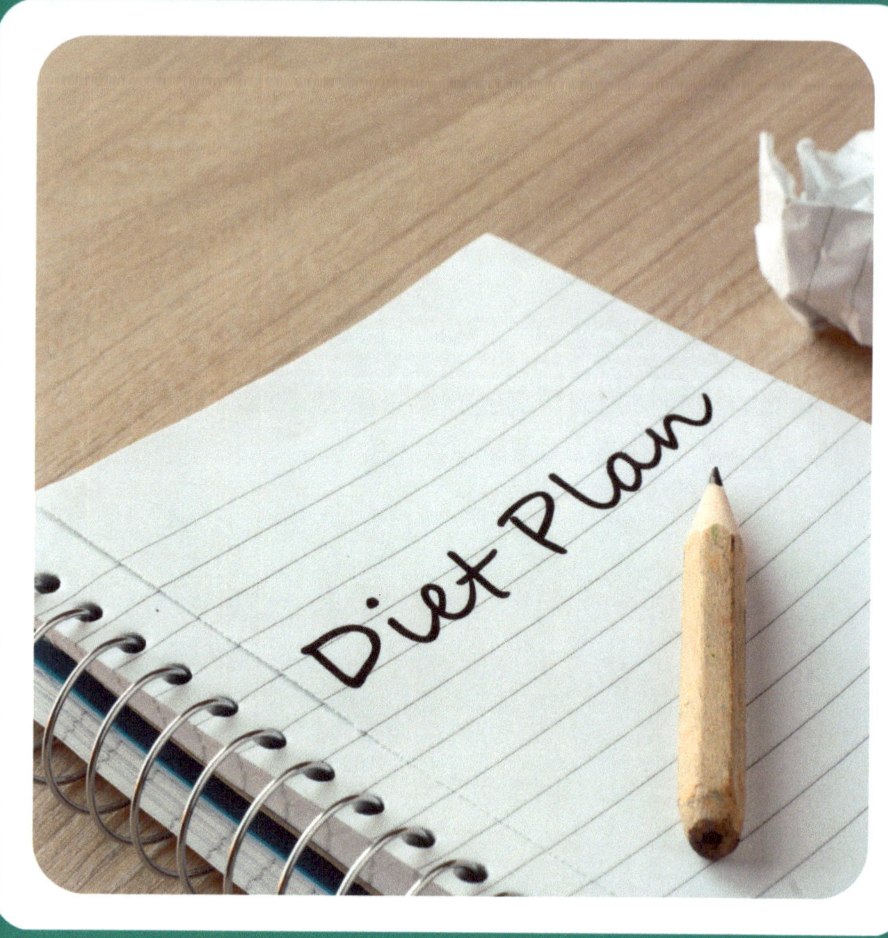

DIET CHART OF PROPHET MUHAMMAD PBUH

It is important to note that there is no single diet chart for Prophet Muhammad (peace be upon him) that has been recorded in detail. However, there are certain practices and habits that he followed which can serve as a guideline for a healthy diet.

Prophet Muhammad (peace be upon him) practiced moderation in his eating habits and emphasized the importance of a balanced diet. He often fasted on Mondays and Thursdays, as well as during the month of Ramadan. He also encouraged his followers to eat slowly and in moderation, avoiding overeating.

In terms of specific foods, Prophet Muhammad (peace be upon him) enjoyed dates and would often break his fast with them. He also ate vegetables such as cucumber, eggplant, and pumpkin, as well as meat such as lamb, chicken, and beef. He preferred to eat lean meat and would sometimes eat fish as well.

Prophet Muhammad (peace be upon him) was also known to drink plenty of water, and encouraged his followers to do the same. He would often drink water before and after meals, and would also drink milk and honey.

It is important to note that Prophet Muhammad (peace be upon him) did not have access to the same variety and abundance of food that we have today. In times of hardship, he would survive on very little food and water, relying on the blessings of Allah for sustenance. Despite this, he remained physically fit and healthy throughout his life.

In summary, a healthy diet in the light of Prophet Muhammad's (peace be upon him) practices would consist of a balance of whole grains, lean proteins, vegetables, fruits, and plenty of water. Eating in moderation and avoiding overeating is also emphasized.

HONEY

Honey is a natural sweetener and medicinal substance that has been used for thousands of years. It has antioxidant, antibacterial properties, and is mentioned in the Quran for its healing properties.

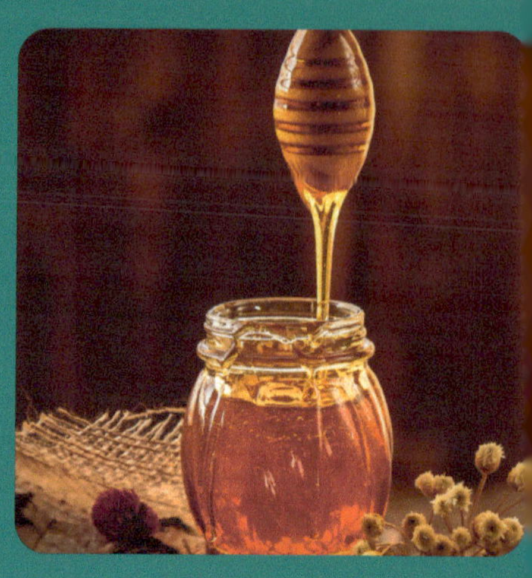

HALAL MEAT

Halal meat refers to meat that is prepared and consumed according to Islamic dietary laws. The process involves slaughtering the animal in a specific manner and reciting a prayer, ensuring that the meat is permissible for Muslims to eat.

PUMPKIN

Pumpkin is a nutrient-dense and versatile vegetable, enjoyed by Prophet Muhammad (peace be upon him) and recommended for its health benefits. It can be used in a variety of dishes, from sweet to savory.

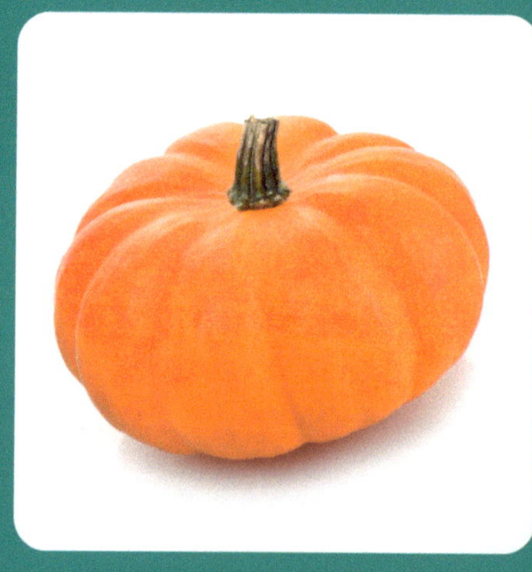

EXERCISE AND FITNESS IN ISLAM

Islam places great emphasis on taking care of one's physical health and well-being. Physical fitness is not only a means of maintaining a healthy body but also a way to strengthen one's connection with Allah (SWT). There are several Quranic verses and Hadiths that encourage Muslims to stay physically active and engage in various forms of exercise.

One of the most significant benefits of exercise in Islam is that it helps maintain a sound mind and body. In the Quran, Allah (SWT) says, "And whoever strives only strives for [the benefit of] himself. Indeed, Allah is free from need of the worlds." (29:6) This verse highlights the importance of striving to improve oneself physically, mentally, and spiritually. Regular exercise not only improves physical fitness but also helps reduce stress, anxiety, and depression, leading to a healthier and more balanced lifestyle.

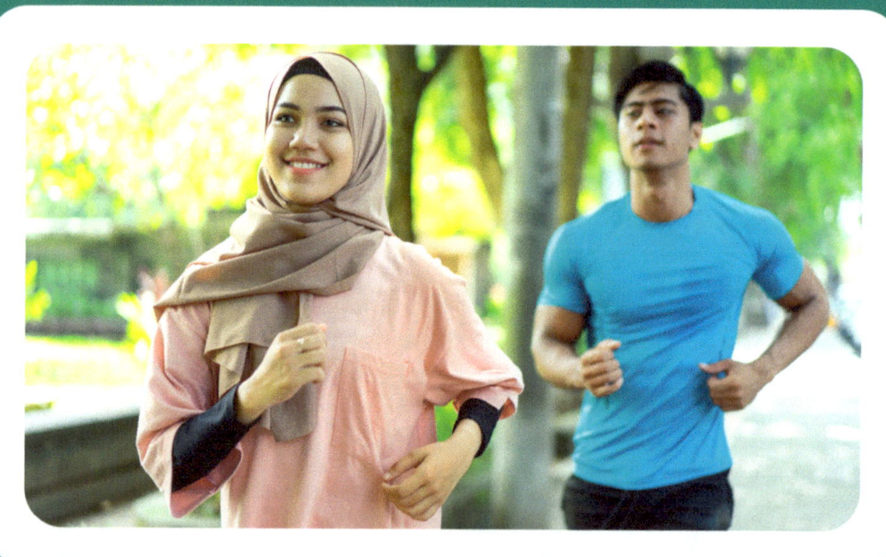

Prophet Muhammad (peace be upon him) was a strong advocate of physical fitness and encouraged his companions to engage in different types of exercise. One of the most popular forms of exercise in Islam is walking, which was a favorite of Prophet Muhammad (peace be upon him). He used to walk for long distances, both for the purpose of worship and daily activities. According to a Hadith, Prophet Muhammad (peace be upon him) once said, "The feet of a person will not move on the Day of Judgment until he is asked about four things: his life - how he spent it, his knowledge - how he acted upon it, his wealth - where he earned it and how he spent it, and his body - how he used it." This Hadith emphasizes the importance of taking care of one's body, which includes engaging in physical exercise.

In addition to walking, other types of permissible exercises in Islam include swimming, horseback riding, archery, and sword fighting. These activities not only promote physical fitness but also provide an opportunity for Muslims to learn and practice important life skills.

It is essential to note that exercise in Islam should be done in moderation and with the intention of pleasing Allah (SWT). One should not engage in any form of exercise that may lead to harm or injury to oneself or others. It is also recommended to seek the advice of a qualified medical professional before starting any new exercise routine.

In conclusion, physical fitness and exercise are integral parts of Islam and play a vital role in maintaining a healthy mind and body. Muslims are encouraged to engage in various forms of permissible exercise regularly and with the intention of pleasing Allah (SWT). By taking care of our bodies we can better serve Allah (SWT) and fulfill our duties as Muslims.

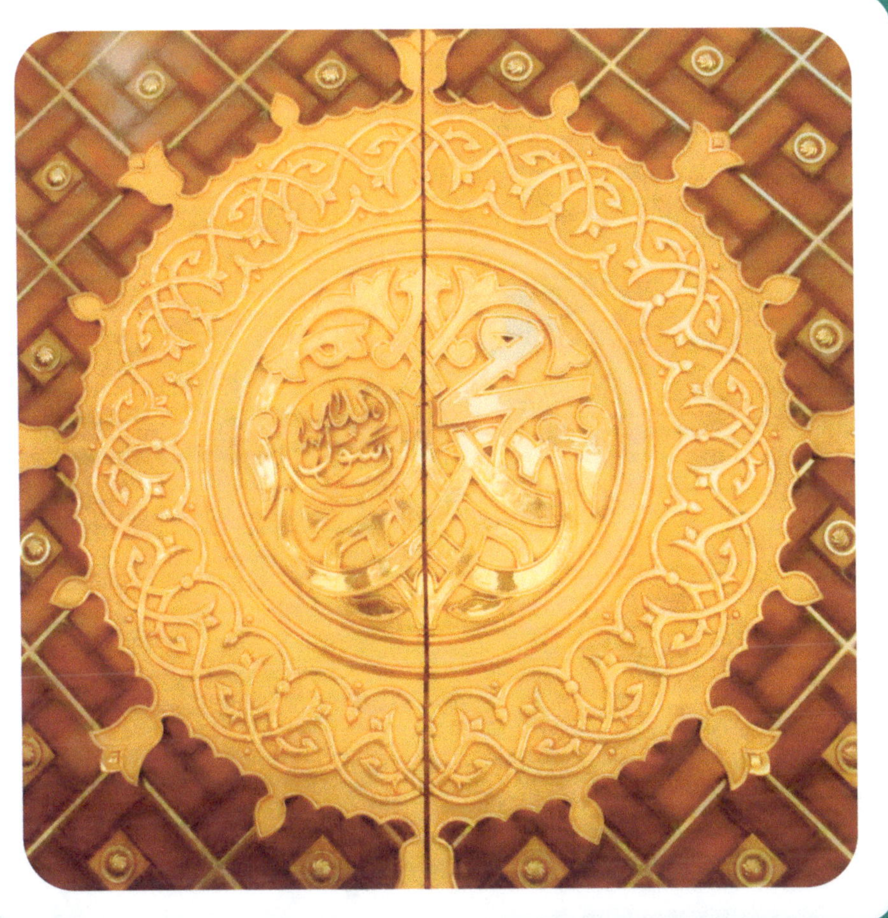

PROPHET MUHAMMAD'S (PBUH) FITNESS HABITS IN ISLAM

Prophet Muhammad (pbuh) emphasized the importance of physical fitness and encouraged his companions to engage in regular exercise. He led by example and participated in various physical activities himself. He would often race with his wife Aisha (may Allah be pleased with her) and engage in other sports like archery and horseback riding.

Prophet Muhammad (pbuh) also encouraged his companions to engage in physical exercise and take care of their bodies. He advised them to engage in activities like swimming, wrestling, and horse riding, and to maintain a healthy diet. He even prescribed certain exercises for specific ailments and recommended them to his companions.

On several occasions, Prophet Muhammad (pbuh) demonstrated the importance of physical fitness and endurance. During the Battle of Uhud, he climbed to the top of a mountain to encourage his companions and remained there for a considerable time, despite being injured. Similarly, during the Battle of the Trench, he helped his companions dig the trench, and even carried heavy stones to strengthen it.

Prophet Muhammad (pbuh) also emphasized the importance of consistency in exercise and physical activity. He advised his companions to engage in regular physical activity and not to overexert themselves. He encouraged them to maintain a balanced approach to exercise and fitness and not to neglect other aspects of their lives, such as spiritual and mental health.

Overall, the example of Prophet Muhammad (pbuh) demonstrates the importance of physical fitness in Islam and the need for Muslims to take care of their bodies. His teachings emphasize the importance of balance and consistency in exercise and the need for a healthy diet.

CHAPTER 4

FITNESS OF KIDS IN ISLAM

Physical fitness is important for everyone, regardless of age. However, it is especially important for children as they are still developing physically and mentally. In Islam, the importance of physical fitness for kids is highlighted through various teachings in the Quran and Hadith.

One of the main principles emphasized in Islam is the concept of balance and moderation. This applies to all aspects of life, including physical fitness. As parents and caregivers, it is important to encourage children to engage in physical activity that is appropriate for their age and abilities, while also ensuring they are not overexerting themselves or neglecting other important aspects of their lives such as education and socialization.

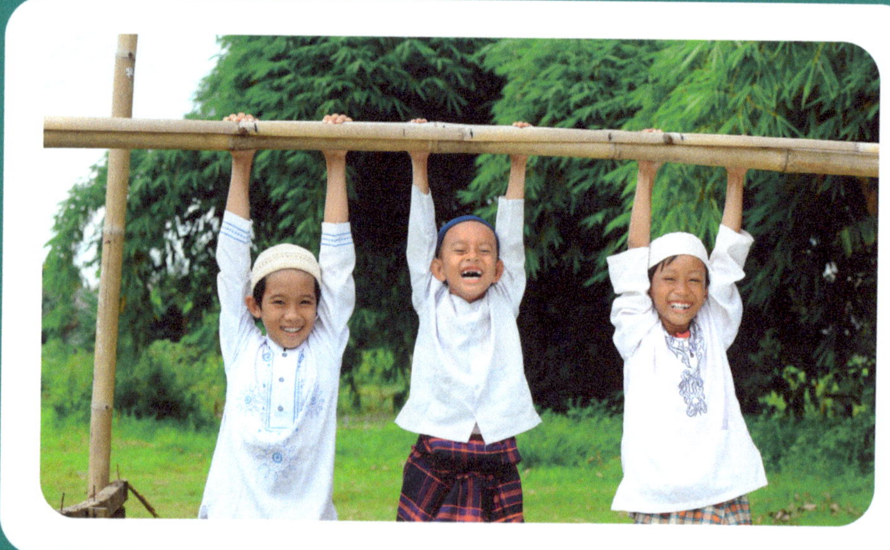

There are many physical activities and exercises that are appropriate and beneficial for children. Some examples include swimming, cycling, hiking, team sports, and martial arts. These activities not only promote physical fitness, but also help develop important social and cognitive skills, such as teamwork, problem-solving, and self-discipline.

In addition to physical activity, a balanced and nutritious diet is also crucial for children's physical fitness and overall health. The Quran encourages the consumption of wholesome and pure foods and discourages overeating or consuming foods that are harmful to the body. Parents and caregivers should aim to provide their children with a healthy and balanced diet, while also teaching them the importance of mindful eating and moderation.

Prophet Muhammad (PBUH) also emphasized the importance of physical fitness and healthy habits for children. He encouraged parents to teach their children to ride horses, swim, and engage in archery. These activities not only promote physical fitness but also help develop important life skills and character traits such as courage, perseverance, and self-discipline.

Prophet Muhammad (PBUH) also stressed the importance of being mindful of children's physical limitations and abilities. He is reported to have said, "Your children have rights over you, and one of those rights is that you teach them to swim, to ride, and to shoot." This emphasizes the importance of providing children with opportunities to engage in physical activity, but also ensuring that it is appropriate and safe for their age and abilities.

Overall, physical fitness for kids is an important aspect of Islamic teachings. Parents and caregivers have a responsibility to ensure that children are engaging in appropriate physical activity, while also promoting balance and moderation in all aspects of their lives. By following the guidance of the Quran and Hadith, and emulating the habits of Prophet Muhammad (PBUH), we can help children develop physically, mentally, and spiritually.

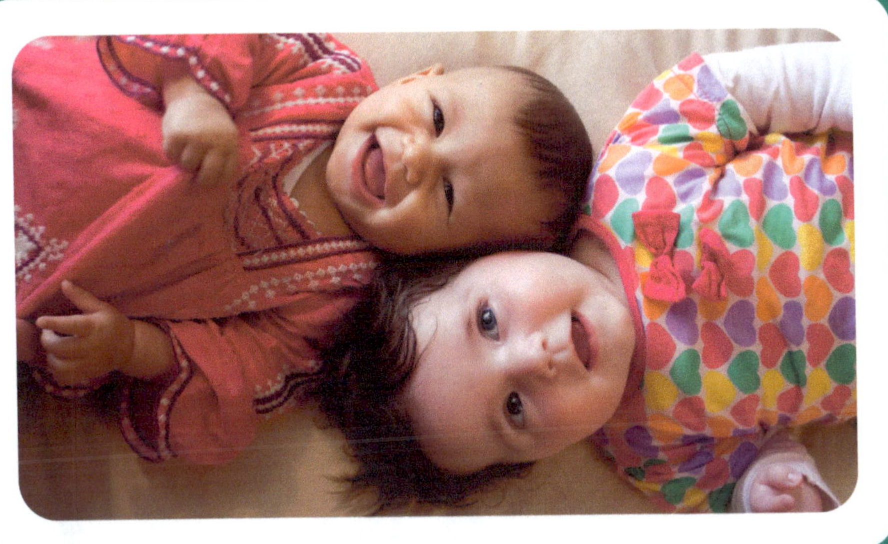

PHYSICAL FITNESS AND ACTIVITIES OF CHILDREN IN ISLAM

In Islam, the physical fitness and health of children are highly valued, and the Sunnah of Prophet Muhammad (PBUH) provides numerous examples of this. The Prophet Muhammad (PBUH) emphasized the importance of physical activity and encouraged children to engage in various exercises and sports, such as swimming, archery, and horse riding. He also taught them the importance of maintaining a healthy diet and getting enough sleep. The Prophet Muhammad (PBUH) himself would regularly engage in physical activities with his own children and grandchildren, setting an excellent example for other Muslim parents and caregivers to follow. By promoting physical fitness for children, we can help them grow up to be healthy, active, and productive members of society.

Prophet Muhammad (PBUH) encouraged physical activity and exercise for children, and it is reported that he would play with his grandchildren, Hassan and Hussain (RA) (may Allah be pleased with them) and engage them in various physical activities such as racing and wrestling. He also taught them to ride horses and camels, swim, and practice archery.

Prophet Muhammad (PBUH) also emphasized the importance of outdoor activities and spending time in nature, and would take his grandchildren on trips and excursions. He encouraged children to participate in games and sports that involve physical activity, such as running, swimming, and ball games.

In addition to these activities, Prophet Muhammad (PBUH) also taught children the importance of discipline and self-control, and encouraged them to engage in activities that promote physical and mental health. He emphasized the importance of balance and moderation in all aspects of life, including physical fitness and exercise, and warned against excessive indulgence in any activity.

Overall, this subtopic provides a comprehensive overview of the physical fitness and activities of children in the Sunnah of Prophet Muhammad (PBUH), and highlights the importance of physical fitness and exercise for children in Islam.

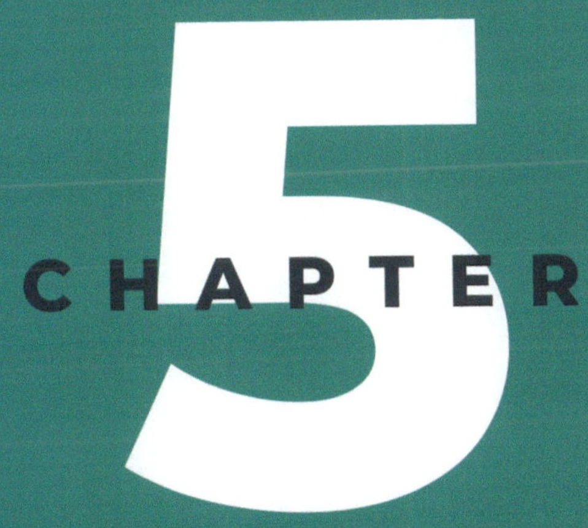

ISLAM AND SPORTS

Sports play an important role in many cultures around the world, and Islam is no exception. Islam encourages physical activity and sportsmanship, as well as teamwork and perseverance. This chapter explores the relationship between Islam and sports, and how Muslim athletes can integrate their faith into their athletic pursuits.

In Islam, physical fitness is considered important not only for health reasons, but also for spiritual reasons. The Prophet Muhammad (peace be upon him) himself engaged in various physical activities, such as swimming, horseback riding, and archery. He also encouraged his companions to participate in physical activity and sports, emphasizing the importance of balance in all aspects of life.

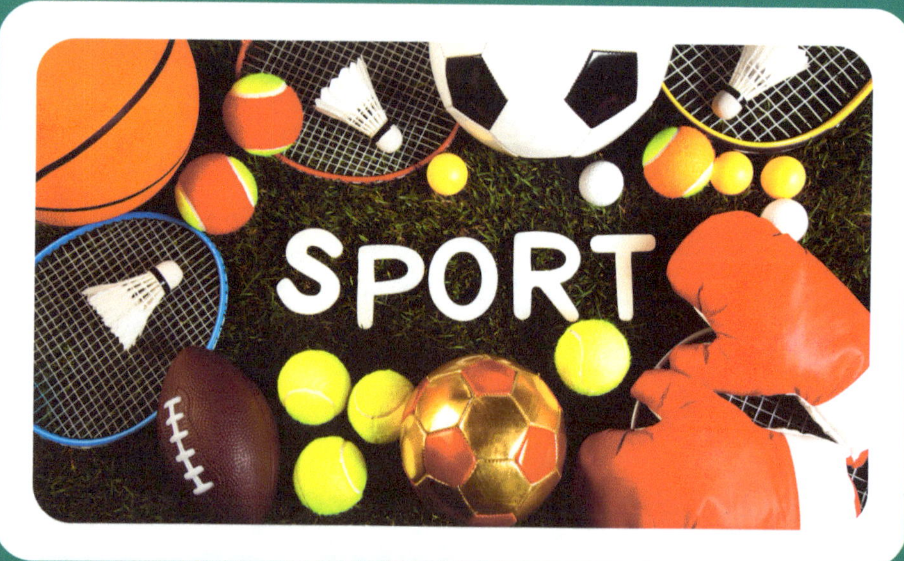

There are many sports that Muslims can participate in, as long as they adhere to Islamic principles of modesty, fairness, and good sportsmanship. Some popular sports among Muslims include soccer, basketball, swimming, and running.

It is also important for Muslim athletes to maintain their religious practices while engaging in sports. This can be achieved through proper scheduling and time management, as well as observing Islamic practices such as prayer and fasting. Muslim athletes should also be mindful of their conduct both on and off the field, adhering to Islamic values of respect and honesty.

In addition to individual sports, Islam also encourages teamwork and community through group sports. The Prophet Muhammad (peace be upon him) himself engaged in team sports such as wrestling and swordplay with his companions. This emphasizes the importance of working together towards a common goal, and supporting one another in achieving that goal.

One important aspect of sports in Islam is to always maintain a balance between physical activity and spiritual well-being. Excessive focus on sports and physical fitness can lead to neglecting one's religious practices, and can also result in arrogance and a lack of humility. Therefore, it is important for Muslim athletes to always prioritize their faith, while still enjoying and benefiting from sports.

In conclusion, sports and physical activity are important in Islam, as long as they are pursued within the boundaries of Islamic principles and values. Muslim athletes can use sports as a means of strengthening their physical and spiritual health while also building teamwork and community. By maintaining a balance between sports and spiritual well-being, Muslims can achieve a well-rounded and fulfilling lifestyle.

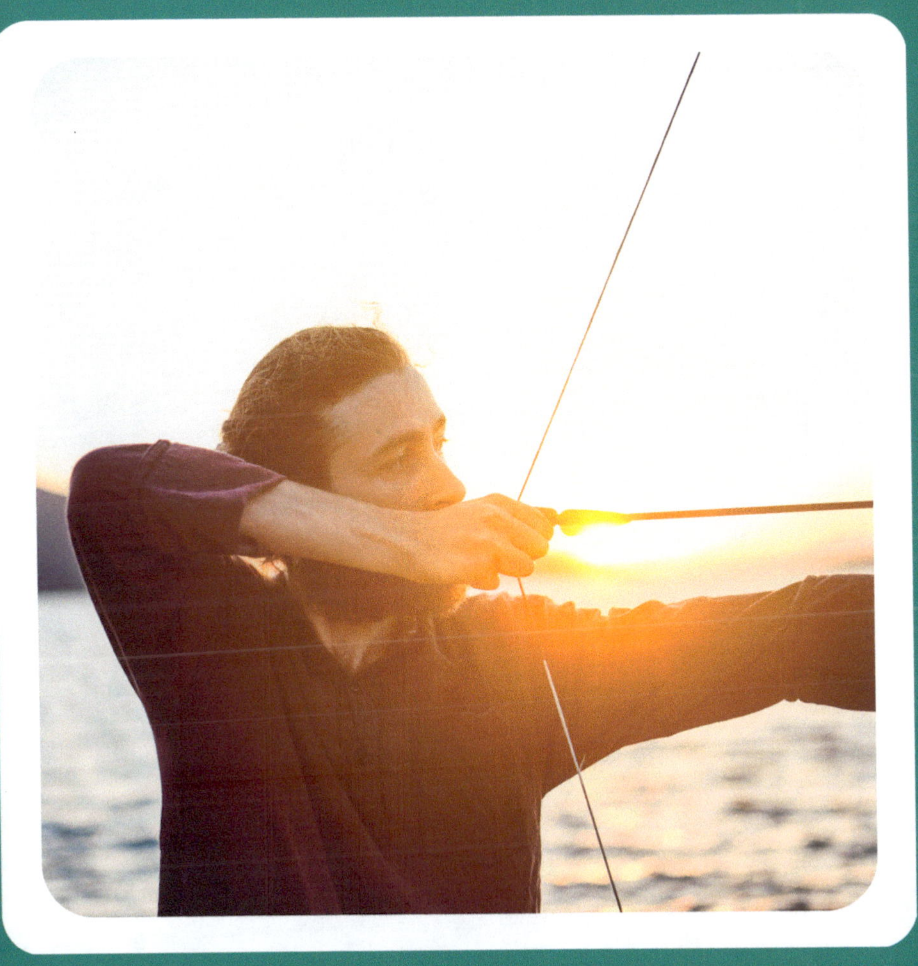

HISTORY AND IMPORTANCE OF SPORTS IN ISLAM

The history of sports in Islam is rich and diverse, with physical activity and sports being highly encouraged in the Islamic faith. The Prophet Muhammad (peace be upon him) himself was known to participate in various physical activities and encouraged his followers to do the same.

In fact, many of the early Muslims were skilled in various forms of physical activity and sports. Archery, horseback riding, swimming, and wrestling were among the popular sports during the time of the Prophet.

In Islam, physical fitness is seen as an essential component of overall well-being, and the Quran encourages Muslims to take care of their bodies and strive for balance in all aspects of their lives. This includes engaging in physical activity and sports.

Furthermore, Islam promotes sportsmanship and fair play, emphasizing the importance of treating opponents with respect and dignity. The Prophet Muhammad (peace be upon him) taught that one who cheats or deceives in sports has betrayed their faith.

Today, many Muslim athletes participate in sports at both the amateur and professional levels, representing their countries and communities with pride. Islamic countries also host many international sporting events, such as the Olympics, and have made significant contributions to the development of sports and physical activity around the world.

In conclusion, the history of sports in Islam is rich and diverse, with physical activity and sports being highly encouraged in the Islamic faith. The importance of maintaining physical fitness and engaging in sportsmanship is emphasized in the Quran and the teachings of the Prophet Muhammad (peace be upon him). Muslim athletes continue to excel in various sports around the world, reflecting the values and principles of their faith.

CHAPTER 6

MENTAL HEALTH AND WELL-BEING IN ISLAM

Mental health is a vital component of overall well being, and Islam emphasizes the importance of taking care of one's mental health. This chapter explores the significance of mental health and well being in Islam and the various ways in which Islamic principles can be applied to promote relaxation and stress management.

One of the central principles of Islam is the importance of achieving balance in all aspects of life including mental and emotional health. In the Quran, Allah reminds us that He does not burden a soul beyond its capacity and encourages us to seek His help and guidance during times of hardship. This reminds us that mental health issues are not a sign of weakness or failure but rather a natural part of the human experience.

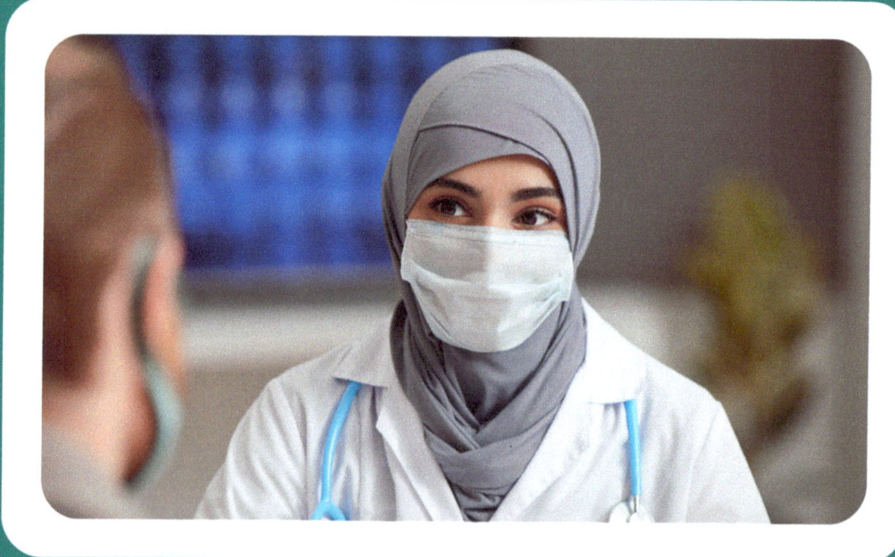

n addition to seeking Allah's help, Islam also provides practical strategies for managing stress and promoting mental well-being. These strategies include regular prayer, meditation, and seeking knowledge about the religion. Islam also encourages social support and community engagement, which can be helpful in times of stress and difficulty.

Another way in which Islam promotes mental well-being is through the concept of gratitude. Gratitude is a central theme in the Quran and Hadith, and practicing gratitude has been shown to have a positive impact on mental health. Islam encourages us to be grateful for the blessings in our lives, both big and small, and to recognize that every difficulty we face is an opportunity to grow and learn.

Finally, Islam recognizes the importance of seeking professional help when needed. While seeking help from Allah and implementing Islamic principles can be beneficial, it is also important to seek out medical and psychological assistance when necessary. Islam encourages us to take care of our bodies and minds and to seek help when we need it.

In conclusion, mental health and well-being are essential components of the Islamic way of life. By seeking Allah's help, implementing Islamic principles, practicing gratitude, and seeking professional help when needed, Muslims can take care of their mental health and promote overall well-being.

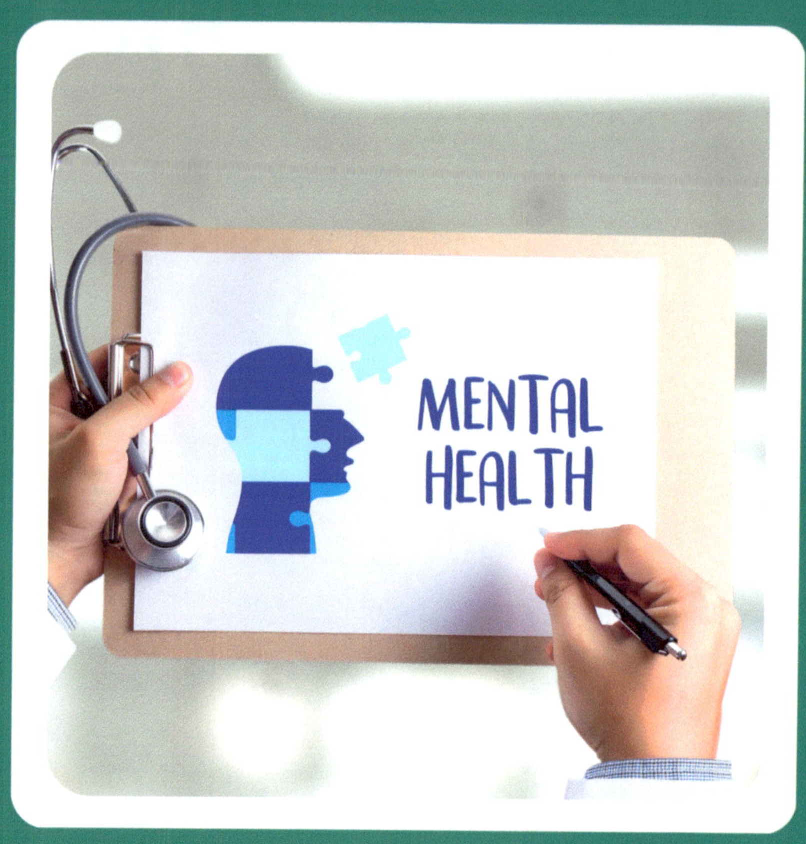

PROMOTING MENTAL HEALTH AND WELL-BEING THROUGH ISLAMIC PRACTICES

Islam emphasizes the importance of mental health and well-being, and provides numerous ways for individuals to maintain and improve their mental health through various practices. One of the most effective ways is through the power of dua and supplications, which involve asking Allah for guidance, forgiveness, and protection.

Prayer (salah) is also a significant aspect of Islamic practice that can promote mental health and well-being. Through performing salah, individuals can find inner peace, reduce stress and anxiety, and develop a deeper connection with Allah.

Fasting during Ramadan is another practice that can help in promoting mental health and well-being. By abstaining from food and drink during the day, individuals can learn self-discipline, self-control, and patience, which are valuable skills for maintaining good mental health.

Reading the Quran, doing dhikr and tasbeeh of Allah's attributes, and reciting masnoon duas and sunnah duas can also be effective ways of promoting mental health and well-being. These practices can provide comfort, calmness, and clarity of mind, and help individuals to overcome negative thoughts and emotions.

Finally, listening to Quran recitation with or without translation can also be an effective way of promoting mental health and well-being. The soothing and calming effect of Quran recitation can help individuals to relax and reduce stress, and gain a deeper understanding and connection with Allah.

Overall, Islam provides various practices that can promote mental health and well-being. By incorporating these practices into our daily lives, we can maintain good mental health, and find inner peace, happiness, and contentment in our lives.

PHYSICAL FITNESS FOR WOMEN IN ISLAM

Physical fitness is important for everyone, including Muslim women. However, there are certain guidelines and principles that Muslim women should follow when engaging in physical activities to ensure that they maintain their modesty and uphold Islamic values.

One important principle for Muslim women is to dress modestly when engaging in physical activities. This means covering the body appropriately in loose-fitting clothing that does not reveal the shape of the body. Muslim women can wear sport hijabs, long-sleeved tops, and loose-fitting pants or skirts that cover their legs. This will not only help them maintain their modesty but also provide comfort and ease during physical activities.

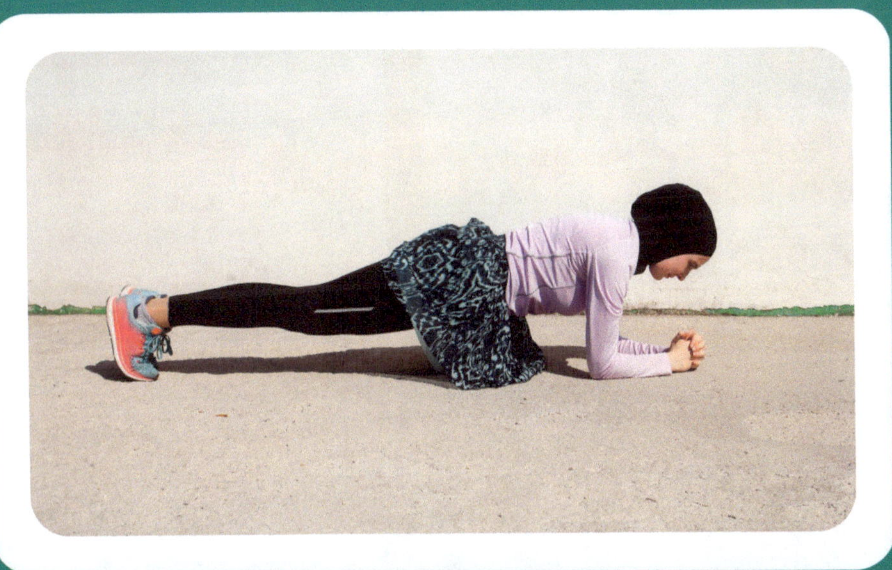

In addition to dressing modestly, Muslim women should also consider engaging in physical activities that are appropriate for their gender and physical capabilities. Islam encourages women to engage in physical activities that are beneficial for their overall health and well-being, but also take into consideration their unique physical needs and limitations. For example, women may prefer activities such as swimming, yoga, or brisk walking that are less physically demanding than weightlifting or other high-intensity workouts.

Furthermore, Muslim women can engage in physical activities that also have spiritual benefits. For instance, they can participate in group exercise classes that incorporate Islamic principles and teachings, such as reciting Quranic verses or making dhikr during breaks. This can help them feel spiritually uplifted and connected to their faith while improving their physical fitness.

Lastly, Muslim women should also prioritize their safety when engaging in physical activities. They should choose safe and secure locations for their workouts, such as gyms or community centers, and exercise with a buddy or in groups when possible. This will not only ensure their physical safety but also provide them with a sense of camaraderie and support during their fitness journey.

In conclusion, physical fitness is an important aspect of a Muslim woman's overall health and well-being. By adhering to Islamic principles of modesty, appropriateness, and safety, Muslim women can engage in physical activities that benefit their physical, emotional, and spiritual health.

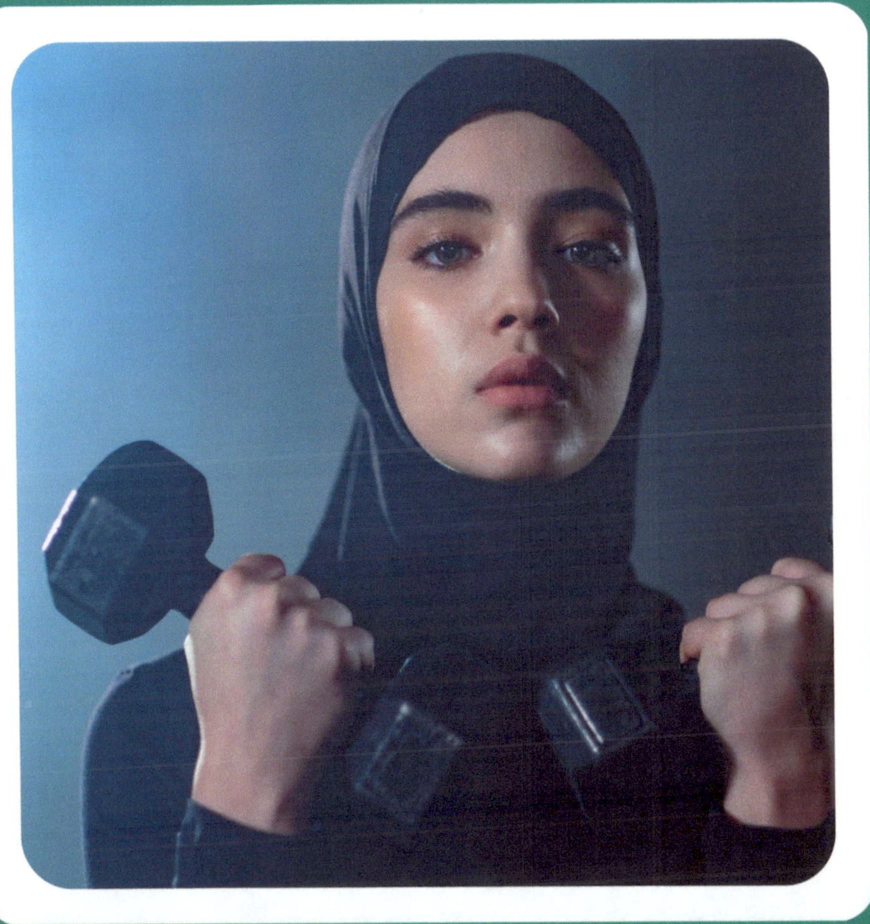

ENCOURAGEMENT FOR WOMEN'S PHYSICAL ACTIVITY IN ISLAM

In Islam, physical activity and exercise are not only encouraged for men but also for women. The Prophet Muhammad (PBUH) emphasized the importance of women's physical fitness and encouraged them to engage in activities that would keep them healthy and fit.

The Prophet (PBUH) would often advise women to participate in physical activities such as swimming, archery, and horse riding. He also encouraged women to engage in household chores that require physical effort, such as grinding grain, carrying water, and weaving. In doing so, the Prophet (PBUH) taught women that physical activity and exercise are important for their physical and mental health.

In addition to physical activities, the Prophet (PBUH) also encouraged women to maintain a healthy and balanced diet. He advised them to eat nutritious foods such as dates, honey, and milk, and to avoid foods that are harmful to their health.

Furthermore, the Prophet (PBUH) taught that women should dress modestly while engaging in physical activity and exercise. This includes wearing loose-fitting clothing that covers the body appropriately, as well as a headscarf for Muslim women.

In summary, the Prophet Muhammad (PBUH) recognized the importance of physical fitness and exercise for women in Islam. He encouraged women to participate in physical activities that are beneficial for their health and well-being, while also emphasizing the importance of maintaining modesty in the process.

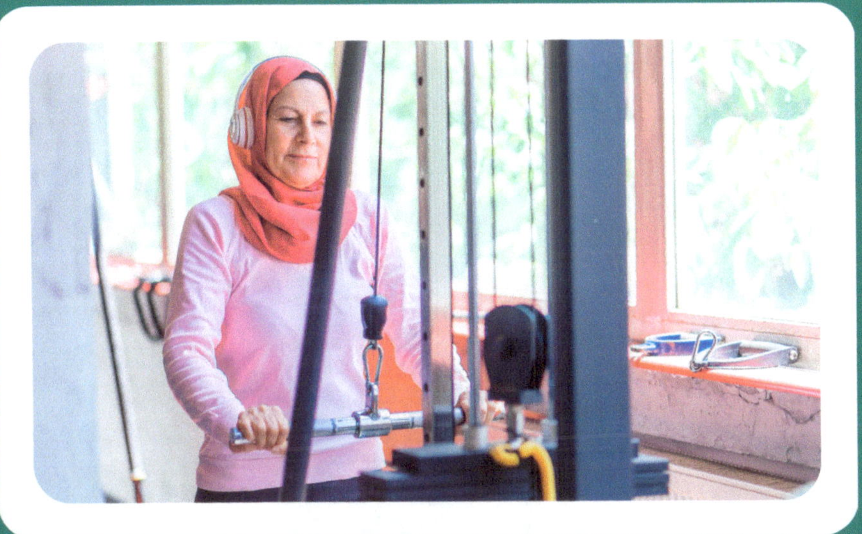

WOMEN'S MODESTY AND EXERCISE IN ISLAM

Muslim women are encouraged to prioritize their physical fitness and engage in appropriate exercises for their well-being. However, it is important to note that Islamic principles of modesty dictate that women should not exercise in front of men who are not their mahram (close male relatives). This is to protect women's privacy and preserve their modesty, as well as to avoid any potential for inappropriate interactions. Prophet Muhammad (peace be upon him) emphasized the importance of modesty and encouraged women to exercise in private or in the company of other women. There are many exercises and physical activities that women can do in the privacy of their own homes or in all-female spaces, such as yoga, Pilates, swimming, and even weightlifting. It is important for Muslim women to prioritize their physical health while also upholding the values of modesty and privacy in Islam.

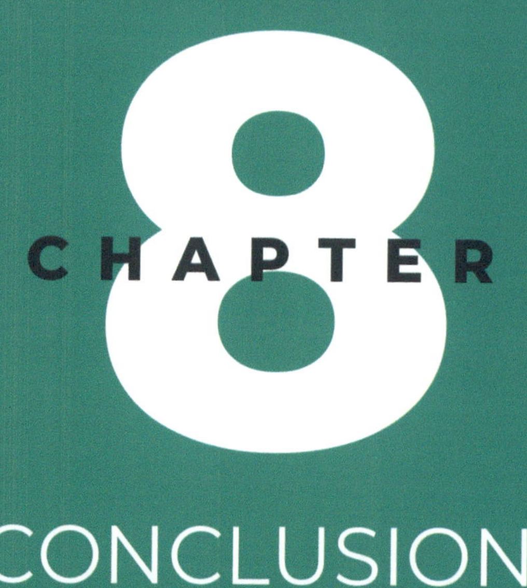

CHAPTER 8

CONCLUSION

Physical fitness is an essential component of a healthy and balanced lifestyle, and it is no different in Islam. Throughout this book, we have explored the Quranic and Hadith-based principles for physical fitness, discussed the importance of maintaining a balanced diet, and delved into the various forms of physical exercise and activity that are permissible in Islam.

Islam emphasizes the importance of maintaining good health and taking care of our bodies. Allah SWT says in the Quran, "And spend in the way of Allah and do not throw [yourselves] with your [own] hands into destruction [by refraining]." (2:195) This verse teaches us that we should not neglect our health and well-being and that we should take care of ourselves in order to better serve Allah and our community.

Prophet Muhammad (PBUH) also emphasized the importance of physical fitness and exercise for both men and women. He encouraged his companions to engage in physical activity and sports, and he himself would engage in physical labor and exercise. He also encouraged women to exercise and engage in physical activity within the bounds of modesty and with proper hijab.

Furthermore, Prophet Muhammad (PBUH) taught us the importance of moderation in all aspects of life, including our diet and exercise. He said, "The most beloved of deeds to Allah are those that are consistent, even if they are small." (Sahih Bukhari)

In conclusion, physical fitness is an integral part of our overall well-being, and it is essential for us to maintain a balanced and healthy lifestyle in accordance with Islamic principles. By following the guidance of the Quran and Sunnah, we can lead healthy and fulfilling lives, while also serving Allah SWT and our community to the best of our ability.

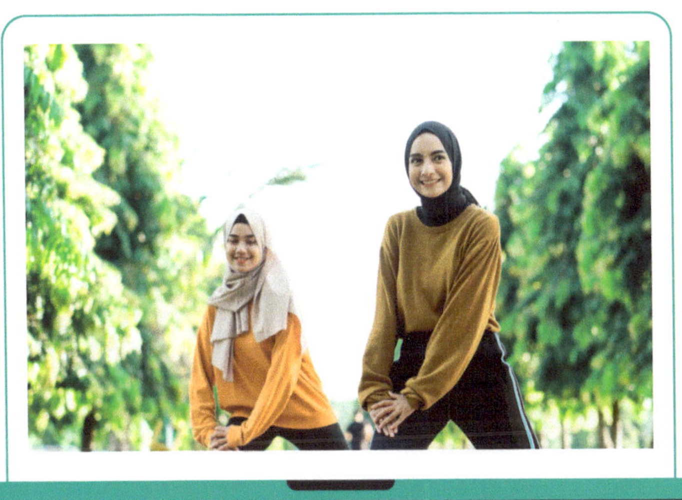

FIT FOR FAITH

Quranic and Hadith-Based Principles for Physical Fitness and Well-being

Fit for Faith is a comprehensive guide that explores the Islamic principles of physical fitness and well-being based on the Quran, Hadith, and Sunnah. This book provides practical guidance on how to incorporate healthy eating habits, regular exercise, and stress management techniques into daily routines, all while staying true to Islamic values and principles. From the importance of maintaining good health to the benefits of a balanced diet and exercise, Fit for Faith provides a holistic approach to physical fitness and well-being in the context of Islam. Whether you are a seasoned fitness enthusiast or just starting your journey towards a healthier lifestyle, Fit for Faith is a must-read for anyone looking to improve their physical and spiritual well-being.

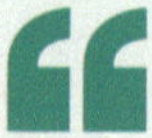

"The strong believer is better and more beloved to Allah than the weak believer, although there is good in both."

Prophet Muhammad (PBUH)
[Sahih Muslim]

www.ingramcontent.com/pod-product-compliance
Lightning Source LLC
Chambersburg PA
CBHW041803260726
48664CB00034B/152